MY WEIGHT OBSESSION
(I wish I was skinny)

Having the right reasons to lose   weight and ways to lose weight effectively

Table of content

<u>*Chapter 1*</u>

<u>***WHAT IS BODY IMAGE***</u>

Body image is the way we view ourselves physically, the way we internally and externally talk about ourselves based on how we look, the reflection we see in the mirror. Body image is defined as the mental picture one forms of one's body as a whole, including its physical characteristics and one's attitudes towards these characteristics.

What are the four aspects of body
image?
* The way you see your
body is your perceptual
body image....
* The way you feel about
your body is your
affective body image....
* The way you think about
your body is your
  cognitive body image....
* The way you behave or you engage
in as a result of your body
image are your behavioral
body image....

Are we neutral, kind, or mean to ourselves? Do we find ourselves being critical or neutral about the observations we make about our body and appearance? Do we find ourselves making strong judgments about our body that leave us feeling unworthy, less than, or undeserving?How do you feel about your body? What do you see when you look in the mirror? Do you see imperfections? Do you see strength? Do you feel appreciation? How do you feel ? How do you feel ? Do you feel capable?

**How we answer those questions is all part
of our body image.**

How Is 'Body Positivity' Related to Body Image?Yes, the body positivity which is about loving your body and having a positive outlook no matter your shape or size. It is related to body image. Body positivity means having a healthy body image regardless of what you look like,"body positivity," however, is more often traced back to the mid-1990s and the creation of the Body Positive, a nonprofit with the goal of ending "the harmful consequences of negative body image,"It is the MOST HELPFUL

How Is 'Body Neutrality' Related to Body Image?Body neutrality is a different concept."It encourages taking a neutral approach to our bodies, The term reminds us that we do not have to love our body to respect it, to nourish it, listen to its cues, or to have gratitude for what it can do.Body
neutrality is defined as not supporting
the hatred or the love of your body but defining your own beauty.

Embracing body neutrality rather than
body positivity may be a more achievable
goal for people with body image issues
and those struggling with eating disorders. It creates the space to
cultivate an authentic identity that focuses less on the physical
self and more on our core, image issues are more common in
youth and teenage age.The foundation for a positive or negative
body image starts early.

Young kids,adolescents,teenagers young adults are very
impressionable, always seeking love and care.Their body image
is shaped by what they consume in traditional media and on
social media, as well as via the messages they receive regarding
body and appearance from adults, If these messages are positive,
chances are greater that the young person will establish a
positive body image. But that is a wrong route depending on
other people's view, definition and conditions. Set your rules
yourself; your way! .Generally we all want to be loved but do you
love yourself? You want to be called beautiful,good enough?Can
you tell that you are beautiful,good enough and important? It
starts with lovies.

Let's Talk about Body Positive Movement...
It began as a movement to create a space where bodies that have
been marginalized by society could exist. A place where bodies
that didn't fit the conventional mold could come together to
celebrate, learn from, and support each other.

I'm so grateful for this movement as it's allowed me to dive deep into my fatphobia and create more self-acceptance and love for all bodies, including my own. This is so important in our world today, so much so that I wrote a post on Self Love and Why We Need It.

The fat acceptance movement began in the 1960s and aimed to tackle anti-fat bias in society by raising awareness of discrimination directed towards overweight and obese people.

A positive body image means you feel good in your skin, regardless of whether your body meets the definition of what those around you would consider the ideal shape is. It's a feeling of satisfaction about one's body irrespective of the societal ideal being forced at any given time. For example, consider how you would feel if you tried on shorts from last year and they fit more snuggly than you remember. A body positive way to respond would be: 'Wow, I guess I grew this past year, but that's okay. Bodies are made to change and adapt. I'll find some different shorts instead so I can enjoy the summer and feel comfortable."

What Causes Someone to Have a Negative Body Image?Having a negative body image is the opposite of having a positive body image; it's feeling bad or beating yourself up for the way you look. A negative body image can mean being highly critical of yourself physically and being judgmental about yourself to the point that you start to believe an internal dialogue, which in turn impacts the way you view your worth and
value as a person.

Consider the scenario where you're trying on that pair of shorts from last year that no
longer fit. Someone with a negative body image might react to that situation by thinking that they're a failure for gaining weight or for not being as lean as they were in the past.

A negative body image might be traceable
to a person's teenage years, when it may have been impacted by things like weight changes caused by puberty, pressure to look a certain way, social media posts with unattainable body ideals, having parents who were overly concerned about their own weight, or being exposed to sexual objectification, health issues etc. But regardless of any triggers that negative body image issues can be linked back to, it can certainly outlast someone's teenage years. be an issue across the lifespan — teens grow up to be adults who continue to have issues with body image . Adults can also develop a negative body image, especially if they're prone to comparing themselves to others and feel pressure to
meet socially prescribed beauty standards. Studies have shown that women are more likely to struggle with body image than men. An October 2017 article found that men accounted for about 18 percent of study participants with symptoms of disordered eating. specifically high neuroticism were also associated with poor body image, but the researchers found that this link applied
only to women and not men.

How Body Image Bears on Health and well-Being. Having a negative body image can affect both physical and mental health. How Body Image Affects Physical Health One of the most significant mental and medical issues that comes along with having a negative body image is the connection to the risk of developing an eating disorder.

A negative body image can lead to dieting, which can lead to disordered eating and a host of negative health consequences, Not all dieting leads to an eating disorder, of course, but there is plenty of research that has found that it can contribute.The most serious side effects of eating disorders include infertility, heart damage, brain damage, and organ failure.A negative body image can influence other behaviors as well. You can see people who have negative body image engaging in other types of behaviors and activities to try to fix what they perceive to be problematic like maybe smoking or substance abuse to manage weight, or excessive exercise, which can lead to health issues down the road. People with eating disorders are five times more likely than the general population to use alcohol or illicit drugs, and 11 times more likely to become dependent on either alcohol or drugs.

How Body Image Affects Mental Health, body image problems can also lead to mental health problems, particularly if the body image issues have led to disordered eating. Anxiety or depression can develop at the same time as the eating disorder, or before it or after it, there are some connections between depression and bulimia nervosa, as well as between anxiety and anorexia.

Having a negative body image can impact your overall quality of life. A study published in 2016 found that people who reported having a positive body image (measured by a body image scale that evaluated individuals' satisfaction with various body functions and parts of the body) was closely related to quality of life for study participants, all of whom were from Turkey and over the age of 15.

How and Why Social Media Use Affects Body Image

Today, social media is a factor that can have a big effect on someone's body image and how they see themselves. For many people, social media shapes what defines beauty and attractiveness. And there are countless examples of people using social media to define themselves as individuals placing more importance on the body and almost objectifying it.

Social media can lead people to judge themselves harshly, if their bodies don't resemble what they see online. Being bombarded by images on social media can have a negative impact on body image, because in real life nobody will ever live up
to the Photoshopped or perfectly curated ideal they see in their Instagram feeds. That said, the body image conversations on social media aren't all negative. Social media can serve as another mental health

resource when used mindfully and consumed critically.

Body Image and BIPOC Communities

People from BIPOC (Black, Indigenous, and People of Color) communities may have their own body image struggles, including feeling stuck in between mainstream Western beauty standards that glorify fatness and other body
types that are celebrated within their culture, For a study published 2015, a group of 31 African American women, who participated in a series of focus groups, mostly agreed that bodies that are thick, toned and curvy are considered more ideal than the thin standard of beauty for white people. That can lead to some confusion. "BIPOC people are contending not only with mainstream body ideals but also with our cultures' specific body and beauty ideals. Those ideals can be contradictory, leaving BIPOC people feeling left out of one or both standards. These body image issues can be exacerbated by the fact that
People of color often don't see people that look like them in the media.body image problems facing people in BIPOC communities may be brushed aside. BIPOC people also face having our body image struggles belittled or dismissed by those who believe that our cultural backgrounds protect us from anti-fatness.
There is sometimes a narrative that worrying about body image, especially weight, is a white-people problem, one we either don't have the luxury of worrying about because our communities have more urgent needs or one we simply don't need to worry

about because our communities are allegedly more accepting of larger bodies.

Feeling different from others, or potentially inferior, can negatively affect body image.A person who is differently abled or has a chronic illness can experience even greater feelings of 'my body has betrayed me,' something those affected by diet culture and thin idealism already feel when their body

doesn't 'behave as it should' by getting thin or staying thin. How to Adopt a Healthier Body Image Having a positive body image may not come naturally and that's okay.

Few things you can do to improve the way you see yourself, includes the following:

* Notice your body's strengths and abilities, rather than nitpicking your appearance.

* Write down five things you love about your personality and then five things you love about your body. You might say you don't but try to get them.

* Place positive affirmations around your home to remind yourself about your positive qualities.

* Avoid comparing yourself to others.

* Recognize and restructure cognitive distortions that reinforce negative body image. For instance, be realistic about how others are viewing your physical appearance, rather than assuming others are criticizing you behind your back.

* Use positive self-talk, rather than negative self-talk. Tell yourself "I look happy," not "I'm so fat."

* Avoid triggers that set off negative thoughts. Try unfollowing social media accounts, for example, that cause you to feel worse about your body image.

* Don't expect to feel 100 percent great about your body 100 percent of the time. It's almost impossible to be sane around your body and food in this culture . Accept that you're going to have uncomfortable moments, and don't be mad at yourself when you do.

It's when these negative thoughts about your body interfere with daily functioning (for example, if you're engaging in excessive dieting or exercise or avoiding social activities) that it may be time to consider seeking professional help, You have to know that everyone has negative thoughts about how they look from time to time, but when these harmful behaviors are the response to those kinds of thoughts, it's time for professional help to work through it. That internal chatter and the tone you use when thinking or talking about your appearance (the positive and the negative) is all part of your body image.
The increased poor eating habits and body dissatisfaction. Women were more likely than men to report struggling with eating and worsening body image; and nearly 50 percent of those surveyed reported being
more concerned about the way they looked.

Know your worth

Do you know your value?

But what exactly is knowing your value?
Is it having positive self-esteem?Is it knowing your worth and being able to identify all of your positive qualities? Or is it the way others treat you?No matter how you define it, there are definite ways in which you can identify and also grow your value and self-worth. Check out the following list:

1. _Maintain Positive Self-esteem_

Be comfortable with who you are?! your weight, height, color, status and everything that makes and represents you. Be confident in the work you deliver and your sense of professionalism. No matter how adverse the external situations are, you can always have a sense of inner balance and tranquility.

2. _Recognize The Difference You Make_

Confidently approach a negotiation with full belief in your knowledge, skills, and experience and the difference you can make. Avoid running after quantity but focus more on quality. In the end, it is about the impact and the difference
that you make.

3. *Be Clear About Your Values*

Know your boundaries. Be clear about what behavior, how you like to be treated and spoken to, and you speak out when necessary. Build a character out of values,
not valuables. Define your values and avoid any compromise, be at stake.

4. *Do Not Undercharge For Your Services*

Quite often out of fear of losing business or the desire to win more business, people will undercharge for their services. This is a classic situation where they end up doing much more than they're paid to do. This can set a precedent that could be hard to remove. Just don't charge for the work that the client expects you to do, but for you that you'll add to that work.

5. *See Yourself As A Peer*

Have a personal sense of value and deservedness and assert yourself as
an equal in personal and business
relationships. Nurture and elevate
the best in yourself. Whatever ; never shy away from giving yourself a second
chance.

6. *Engage in work that is exciting and fulfilling*

Commit yourself to your passion.Passionate people are far more creative than one just working to make a living. When you are involved in work that is fulfilling as well as financially rewarding, you are more inclined to work with even greater commitment. Hence, creating a brand value for yourself. You Determine Your Value . It is not for someone else to decide your value but your thoughts, emotions, and most importantly, your actions that determine how others perceive your value,this is why you
have to always have a positive mindset.

How do you see yourself

I remember as a person while growing up I will always look at the mirror and my eye will be filled with tears and I will always break those mirrors that showed me my hurtful image (funny),I had so many scars from cutting my wrist I was so inconsistent with my weight today fat tomorrow skinny and I was always reminded of that from family and friends.but acceptance is key.

Chapter 2

REAL REASON YOU SHOULD LOSE WEIGHT

What is fat anyway?

First, it's worth noting that measuring body size is more arbitrary than it might seem. BMI is used to define "normal," "overweight" and "obese" categories, but it's a flawed metric that was never intended to be used for individuals in the first place, let alone for every person of every background. Moreover, the categories have shifted over the years: in 1998, the National Institutes of Health abruptly moved the "overweight" and "obesity" cutoff points down to include millions more Americans.

BMI also doesn't account for body composition: the ratio of body fat to muscle, bone and other tissues. Some doctors believe that "excess" body fat, especially belly fat, is the real health issue instead of weight -- having a high BMI isn't so much of an issue, they say, if the pounds are mostly muscle.

But how much body fat is too much? Adipose tissue (the technical term for fat) is a crucial component of your bodily systems, from your immune system to your brain health. It stores energy and insulates the body in cold weather. It stores essential fat-soluble vitamins, including vitamins A, E, D and K, which is part of why fatty foods like avocados and nuts are now considered "healthy." And fat also affects your health in other, surprising ways.

Fat people are less likely to die from certain conditions. One of the main reasons that doctors discourage fatness is because higher BMIs are associated with a greater risk of chronic conditions like diabetes, heart disease and heart failure. But there's another important piece of the puzzle.

Metabolic syndrome

Metabolic syndrome is a group of conditions that increase your risk for heart disease, diabetes, and stroke. To be diagnosed with metabolic syndrome, metabolic syndrome is closely linked to overweight and obesity and to a lack of physical activity. Healthy lifestyle changes that help you control your weight may help you prevent and reduce metabolic syndrome.

Breathing problems

Overweight and obesity can also affect how well your lungs work, and excess weight increases your risk for breathing problems.

Sleep apnea

Sleep apnea is a common problem that can happen while you are sleeping. If you have sleep apnea, your upper airway becomes blocked, causing you to breathe irregularly or even stop breathing altogether for short periods of time. Untreated sleep apnea may raise your risk for developing many health problems, including heart disease and diabetes.

Asthma

Asthma is a chronic, or long-term, condition that affects the airways in your lungs. The airways are tubes that carry air in and out of your lungs. If you have asthma, the airways can become inflamed and narrow at times. You may wheeze, cough, or feel tightness in your chest. Obesity can increase your risk of developing asthma, experiencing worse symptoms, and having a harder time managing the condition. Losing weight can make it easier for you to manage your asthma. For people who have severe obesity, weight-loss surgery also called metabolic and bariatric surgery may improve asthma symptoms.

High blood pressure

Overweight and obesity may raise your risk for high blood pressure. High blood pressure, also called hypertension, is a condition in which blood flows through your blood vessels with a force greater than normal. Having a large body size may increase blood pressure because your heart needs to pump harder to supply blood to all your cells. Excess fat may also damage your kidneys, which help regulate blood pressure.

High blood pressure can strain your heart, damage blood vessels, and raise your risk of heart attack, stroke, kidney disease, and death. Losing enough weight to reach a healthy body mass index range may lower high blood pressure and prevent or control related health problems.

Heart disease

Heart disease is a term used to describe several health problems that affect your heart, such as a heart attack, heart failure, angina , or an abnormal heart rhythm. Having overweight or obesity increases your risk of developing conditions that can lead to heart disease, such as high blood pressure, high blood cholesterol , and high blood glucose. In addition, excess weight can also make your heart have to work harder to send blood to all the cells in your body. Losing excess weight may help you lower these risk factors for heart disease.

Stroke

A stroke happens when a blood vessel in your brain or neck is blocked or bursts, cutting off blood flow to a part of your brain. A stroke can damage brain tissue and make you unable to speak or move parts of your body. Overweight and obesity are known to increase blood pressure and high blood pressure is the leading cause of strokes. Losing weight may help you lower your blood pressure and other risk factors for stroke, including high blood glucose and high blood cholesterol.

Fatty liver diseases

Fatty liver diseases develop when fat builds up in your liver, which can lead to severe liver damage, cirrhosis, or even liver failure. These diseases include nonalcoholic fatty liver disease (NAFLD) and nonalcoholic steatohepatitis (NASH).
NAFLD and NASH most often affect people who are overweight or obese. People who have insulin resistance, unhealthy levels of fat in the blood, metabolic syndrome, type 2 diabetes, and certain genes can also develop NAFLD and NASH.

If you are overweight or obese, losing at least 3% to 5% of your body weight may reduce fat in the liver.

Some cancers

Cancer is a collection of related diseases. In all types of cancer, some of the body's cells begin to grow abnormally or out of control. The cancerous cells sometimes spread to other parts of the body.
Overweight and obesity may raise your risk of developing certain types of cancer . Men with overweight or obesity are at a higher risk for developing cancers of the colon , rectum, and prostate. Among women with overweight or obesity, cancers of the breast, lining of the uterus , and gallbladder are more common. Different types of cancer are associated with overweight and obesity. These cancers are: thyroid, breast (postmenopausal women), liver, gallbladder, upper stomach, pancreas, colon and rectum, ovary, endometrium (cancer in the tissue lining the uterus), kidney, multiple myeloma (cancer of blood cells),

adenocarcinoma of the esophagus, and meningioma (cancer in the tissue covering the brain and spinal cord).

Overweight and obesity may increase risk of developing many types of cancer.

Adults who gain less weight as they get older have lower risks of many types of cancer, including colon, kidney, breast, and ovarian cancers.

Osteoarthritis

Having overweight or obesity may raise your risk of getting osteoarthritis by putting extra pressure on your joints and cartilage. If you have excess body fat, your blood may have higher levels of substances that cause inflammation. Inflamed joints may raise your risk for osteoarthritis. Having overweight or obesity may raise your risk of getting osteoarthritis in your knees. If you are overweight or obese, losing weight may decrease stress on your knees, hips, and lower back and lessen inflammation in your body. If you have osteoarthritis, losing weight may improve your symptoms. Research shows that exercise is one of the best treatments for osteoarthritis. Exercise can improve mood, decrease pain, and increase flexibility.

Gout

Gout is a kind of arthritis that causes pain and swelling in your joints. Gout develops when crystals made of a substance called uric acid build up in your joints. Risk factors include having obesity, being male, having high blood pressure, and eating foods high in purines. These foods include red meat, liver, and anchovies.Gout is treated mainly with medicines. Losing weight may also help prevent and treat gout.

Diseases of the gallbladder and pancreas

Overweight and obesity may raise your risk of getting gallbladder diseases, such as gallstones and cholecystitis. People who have obesity may have higher levels of cholesterol in their bile, which can cause gallstones. They may also have a large gallbladder that does not work well. Having a large amount of fat around your waist may raise your risk for developing gallstones. But losing weight quickly also reduces your risk. If you have obesity, talk with your health care professional about how to lose weight safely. Obesity can also affect your pancreas, a large gland behind your stomach that makes insulin and enzymes to help you digest food. People who have obesity have a higher risk of developing inflammation of the pancreas, called pancreatitis. High levels of fat in your blood can also raise your risk of having pancreatitis. You can lower your chances of getting pancreatitis by sticking with a low-fat, healthy eating plan.

Kidney disease

Kidney disease means your kidneys are damaged and can't filter your blood as they should. Obesity raises the risk of developing diabetes and high blood pressure, which are the most common causes of chronic kidney disease (CKD). Even if you don't have diabetes or high blood pressure, having obesity may increase your risk of developing CKD and speed up its progress.If you are overweight or obese, losing weight may help you prevent or delay CKD. If you are in the early stages of CKD, consuming healthy foods and beverages, being active, and losing excess weight may slow the progress of the disease and keep your kidneys healthier longer.

Pregnancy problems

Overweight and obesity raise the risk of developing health problems that can affect the pregnancy and the baby's health.
Pregnant people who have obesity may have a greater chance of developing gestational diabetes, or diabetes that occurs during pregnancy having preeclampsia, or high blood pressure during pregnancy, which can cause severe health problems for the pregnant person and baby if left untreated
needing a caesarean delivery NIH external link or c-section and, as a result, taking longer to recover after giving birth having complications from surgery and anesthesia NIH external link, especially if they have severe obesity gaining more weight or continuing to have overweight or obesity after the baby is born. Having obesity or gaining too much weight during pregnancy can also increase health risks for the baby, including:
- being born larger than expected based on the sex of the baby or the duration of the pregnancy.
- developing chronic diseases as adults, including type 2 diabetes, obesity, heart disease, and asthma.
- Talk with your health care professional about how to reach a healthy weight before pregnancy gain a healthy amount

of weight during pregnancy safely lose weight after your baby is born

Type 2 diabetes

Type 2 diabetes is a disease that occurs when your blood glucose, also called blood sugar, is too high. Nearly 9 in 10 people with type 2 diabetes are overweight or obese. Over time, high blood glucose can lead to heart disease, stroke, kidney disease, eye problems, nerve damage, and other health problems.
If you are at risk for type 2 diabetes, you may be able to prevent or delay diabetes by losing at least 5% to 7% of your starting weight. For instance, if you weigh 200 pounds, your goal would be to lose about 10 to 14 pounds.**Diabetes Risk Management Calculator.** Losing 5% to 7% of your body weight may reduce your risk of diabetes

Fertility problems

Obesity increases the risk of developing infertility . Infertility in women means not being able to get pregnant after a year of trying, or getting pregnant but not being able to carry a pregnancy to term. For men, it means not being able to get a woman pregnant. Obesity is linked to lower sperm count and sperm quality in men. In women, obesity is linked to problems with the menstrual cycle and ovulation. Obesity can also make it harder to become pregnant with the help of certain infertility treatments or procedures. Women with obesity who lose 5% of their body weight may increase their chances of having regular menstrual periods, ovulating, and becoming pregnant.

Sexual function problems

Obesity may also increase the risk of developing sexual function problems. Having overweight or obesity increases the risk of developing erectile dysfunction (ED), a condition in which males are unable to get or keep an erection firm enough for satisfactory sexual intercourse.

Few studies have looked at how obesity may affect female sexual function by contributing to problems such as loss of sexual desire, being unable to become or stay aroused, being unable to have an orgasm, or having pain during sex. But research suggests that healthy eating, increased physical activity, and weight loss may help reduce sexual function problems in people with obesity.

Mental health problems

In addition to increasing the risk for developing physical health problems, obesity can also affect mental health, increasing the risk for developing

long-term stress, body image problems, low self-esteem, depression, eating disorders. Studies show that people with overweight or obesity are also likely to face weight-related bias at school and work, which may cause long-term harm to their quality of life. Losing excess weight has been found to improve body image and self-esteem and reduce symptoms of depression.

But regardless of all this disease being "overweight" might be... good for you?

For years, doctors have believed that the more you weigh, the more unhealthy you are, and the higher your risk of disease and death. But this 2005 study found that people with body mass indexes in the overweight category were actually at lower risk of death than those with a "normal" BMI. This finding alone was surprising enough to land its author, Katherine Flegal, in a "firestorm" of controversy, despite her data being scientifically sound, per Boston Globe. But Flegal wasn't the first researcher to find that weight may influence health in different ways than previously thought. Studies consistently find that overweight or obese individuals with these conditions are less likely to die from them than normal or underweight people, a sign that a high BMI offers some sort of protective effect, another example of the obesity paradox. The phenomenon that fat can offer certain protective health benefits is commonly called the "obesity paradox," a term that shows just how much it flies in the face of everything we thought we knew about fatness and health. "The term 'obesity paradox' is a prime example of weight stigma in the scientific literature," Jeffrey Hunger, an assistant professor of social psychology at Miami University of Ohio told Scientific American in 2020. "Think about it: A paradox is something contradictory or seemingly absurd. This term came about because it was considered absurd that fat people could actually be healthy." But the numbers don't lie. Fat people can be healthy and, in some cases, healthier than those who are thin. Here's what to know.

Fat offers protection from injuries

Having a higher BMI also offers protection from injury in some cases. A 2020 study found that overweight and class I obese trauma patients had better chances of survival than patients with a "normal" BMI. In the past, researchers have also found that subcutaneous fat may help protect from injuries in car crashes in particular, and that overweight people had less severe injuries in a crash than thin people, though the research is mixed on this matter.

Fatness and fitness

It's clear that fat isn't the enemy, and can even be a perk in some cases. But bottom line: There's no need to be thinner in order to be healthy. You can be healthy at any size, while the reverse is also true: one study found that almost half of "overweight" people were metabolically healthy, while 30% of "normal" people were not. Various studies have found that physical activity seems to matter more for health than BMI. In one 2017 study in the Netherlands, for example, people with high BMIs who were very physically active had the same likelihood of heart disease as people with normal BMIs who were just as active. Correlation doesn't equal causation. It's possible that the link between obesity and certain diseases has some other underlying reason. Rather than obesity causing disease, perhaps the two share a common, third cause, such as societal factors or diet. Weight stigma could also play a mediating role in predisposing fat people to illness. Centuries ago, having visible body fat was considered healthy; plumpness was the aspirational beauty standard, not thinness, as detailed in Sabrina Strings' book Fearing the Black Body: The Racial Origins of Fat Phobia. Not only do beauty and health values fluctuate over time, but the very definitions of fatness and thinness are moving goalposts. It's not surprising that being technically "overweight" or "obese" doesn't consistently translate to poorer health . As we age, being "moderately overweight" also seems to offer protection against developing multiple comorbid diseases, making it a "marker of a healthy aging process," according to a 2019 study in Italy. That's in line with Flegal's findings that overweight people live longer. Bigger people tend to be stronger than thin people, according to research, making them better at strength exercises such as weight lifting. That's because, in addition to having more fat tissue, they have more muscle mass, too. This is true for fat people of all ages, from youth to old age.

Chapter 3

WAYS TO LOSE WEIGHT PSYCHOLOGICALLY

Everyone needs a particular diet and exercise to stay fit so Keep that in mind but there are ways to lose weight effectively without much exercise or dieting.Sticking to a conventional diet and exercise plan can be difficult. However, there are several proven tips that can help you eat fewer calories with ease. These are effective ways to reduce your weight, as well as to prevent weight gain in the future.

1. _Chew thoroughly and slow down_
Your brain needs time to process that you've had enough to eat.

Chewing your food thoroughly makes you eat more slowly, which is associated with decreased food intake, increased fullness, and smaller portion sizes. How quickly you finish your meals may also affect your weight. A review of eight studies reported that people who didn't eat quickly had a significantly lower body mass index (BMI) than fast eaters. To get into the habit of eating more slowly, it may help to count how many times you chew each bite. Eating your food slowly can help you feel more full with fewer calories. It is an easy way to lose weight and prevent weight gain.

2. _Use smaller plates for high calorie foods_

The typical food plate is larger today than it was a few decades ago. This trend could contribute to weight gain, since using a smaller plate may help you eat less by making portions look larger. On the other hand, a bigger plate can make a serving look smaller, causing you to add more food. You can use this to your advantage by serving nutrient-dense, lower calorie foods on bigger plates and high calorie foods on smaller plates. Smaller plates can trick your brain into thinking you're eating more than you actually are. Therefore, it's smart to consume higher calorie foods from smaller plates, causing you to eat less.

3. *Eat plenty of protein*

Protein has powerful effects on appetite. It can increase feelings of fullness, reduce hunger, and help you eat fewer calories. This may be because protein affects several hormones that play a role in hunger and fullness, including ghrelin and glucagon-like peptide-1. According to one study in 105 people, those with greater adherence to a high protein diet lost significantly more weight than those who adhered to a standard protein diet. If you currently eat a grain-based breakfast, you may want to consider increasing the protein content of your meals. In one study, people who ate a high protein breakfast with eggs and toast experienced less hunger and ate fewer calories later in the day compared to those who ate a lower protein breakfast with cereal. Some examples of protein-rich foods include chicken breasts, fish, Greek yogurt, lentils, quinoa, and almonds.

Adding protein to your diet has been linked to weight loss and decreased hunger.

4. _**Prepare more meals at home**_

Cooking your own meals at home is a great way to include more nutritious foods in your diet. It might also help promote weight loss. In fact, research suggests that people who prepare more meals at home tend to gain less weight than those who regularly dine out or eat prepared foods.
A 2017 study also found that meal planning may be associated with improved diet quality and a reduced risk of obesity. Try stocking up on nutrient-dense ingredients and experimenting with a few new recipes each week. Preparing more meals at home may help improve the quality of your diet and support weight loss.

5. _**Eat fiber-rich foods**_

Eating fiber-rich foods may increase satiety, helping you feel fuller for longer. Studies also indicate that one type of fiber, viscous fiber, is particularly helpful for weight loss. It increases fullness and reduces food intake. Viscous fiber forms a gel when it comes in contact with water. This gel increases nutrient absorption time and slows down the emptying of your stomach. Viscous fiber is only found in plant foods. Examples include beans, oat cereals, Brussels sprouts, asparagus, oranges, and flax seeds. A weight loss supplement called glucomannan is also very high in viscous fiber, viscous fiber is particularly helpful in reducing appetite and food intake. This fiber forms gel that slows down digestion.

6. ***Drink water regularly***

Drinking water can help you eat less and lose weight, especially if you drink it before a meal. One study found that drinking water before a meal reduced the amount of food consumed, without significantly affecting satiety, Another study showed that drinking 1 pint (568 milliliters) of water before a meal decreased calorie intake and hunger while also increasing fullness and satisfaction If you replace calorie loaded drinks such as soda or juice with water, you may experience an even greater effect. Drinking water before meals may help you eat fewer calories. Replacing a sugary drink with water is particularly beneficial.

7. ***Eat without electronic distractions***

Paying attention to what you eat may help you consume fewer calories. People who eat while they're watching TV or playing computer games may lose track of how much they have eaten. This, in turn, can cause overeating. One 2013 review of 24 studies found that people who were distracted at a meal ate about 10% more in that sitting. Additionally, absent mindedness during a meal has an even greater influence on your intake later in the day. People who were distracted at a meal ate 25% more calories at later meals than those who were present. If you regularly consume meals while watching TV or using electronic devices, you could be inadvertently eating more. These extra calories add up and have a massive impact on your weight in the long term. However, more research is needed, as studies have turned up mixed results on how mindful eating may affect food consumption. People who eat while distracted are more likely to overeat. Paying attention to your meals may help you eat less and lose weight, but more research is needed.

8. *Sleep well and avoid stress*

When it comes to health, people often neglect sleep and stress. Both, in fact, have powerful effects on your appetite and weight. A lack of sleep may disrupt the appetite-regulating hormones leptin and ghrelin. Another hormone, cortisol, becomes elevated when you're stressed
Having these hormones fluctuate can increase your hunger and cravings, leading to higher calorie intake. What's more, chronic sleep deprivation and stress may increase your risk of several diseases, including type 2 diabetes and obesity. Poor sleep and excess stress may imbalance several important appetite regulating hormones, causing you to eat more.

9. *Eliminate sugary drinks*

High consumption of sugar-sweetened beverages, such as soda, has been linked with a higher risk of heart disease and type 2 diabetes. It's very easy to consume excess calories from sugary drinks because liquid calories don't affect fullness the way solid food does. Reducing your intake of sugar-sweetened beverages may be associated with weight loss. According to one meta-analysis, replacing sugar sweetened beverages with low calorie or no calorie sweetened beverages could be linked to reductions in body weight, BMI, and percent body fat. Lower calorie beverage options include water and plain or lightly sweetened coffee or green tea. Sugary drinks have been linked to an increased risk of weight gain and many health conditions. Your brain doesn't register liquid calories as it does solid foods, making you eat more.

The bottom line

Many simple lifestyle habits can help you lose weight. Some have nothing to do with conventional diet or exercise plans.

You can use smaller plates, eat more slowly, drink water, and avoid eating in front of the TV or computer. Prioritizing foods rich in protein and viscous fiber may also help.

However, it's probably best not to try all these things at once. Experiment with one technique for a while, and if that works well for you then try another one.

A few simple changes can have a massive impact on your weight over the long term. Plan a healthy meal. Remember to maintain a good weight do the following, Start today to get in good shape easily

* Walking to get strong. Every fitness trainer will tell you that a balanced workout plan that includes strength, cardio, and flexibility training

* Exotic Veggies

* Sun Bath

* Drink water for fitness

* Count nutrients not calories

* Love your sleep

Don't be deceived, you are more than beautiful because the owner of the universe said so. So don't call him a liar because of your situation.

<u>*Chapter 4*</u>

<u>*MOTIVATE YOURSELF*</u>

<u>*Self-Love, and Body Acceptance*</u>

Body Positive Quotes For Better Body Image I've pulled together some of my favorite body positivity quotes from celebrities, Instagram influencers, authors, and regular people like YOU. Save them for your next bad body image day, share them with your friends or download the graphics and use them to uplift others.

"Feeling beautiful has nothing to do with what you look like." – **Emma WatsonBody**

"Love your body because you only have one."And I said to my body, softly, "I want to be your friend. He took a long breath and replied, "I've been waiting my whole life for this." – **Nayyirah Waheed**

"The best gift you are ever going to give someone the permission to feel safe in their own skin."– **Hannah Brencher**

"Fat is not a bad word."– **Me**

"Loving yourself is the greatest revolution."—**Anna perry**

"That game of comparison you play will strip you of the marvel in your story." – **Ariella Estoria**

"One day I decided that I was beautiful and so I carried out my life as if I was a beautiful girl. It doesn't have anything to do with how the world perceives you. What matters is what you see."
-**Gabourey Sidibe**

"I am a big girl. A voluptuous, curvy, dress-wearing, lesbian. I love my body; it's the only one I'll ever have. I am allowed to look sexy, feel sexy, and be in love. I am worthy of all of those things. And so are you." – **Mary Lambert**

"Confidence is the only key. I can't think of any better representation of beauty than someone who is unafraid to be herself." – **Emma Stone**

"You can be the most beautiful person in the world and everybody sees light and rainbows when they look at you, but if you yourself don't know it, all of that doesn't even matter. Every second that you spend on doubting your worth, every moment that you use to criticize yourself; is a second of your life wasted, is a moment of your life thrown away. It's not like you have forever, so don't waste any of your seconds, don't throw even one of your moments away." – **C. JoyBell C**.

"When you discover your self-worth you will lose interest in anyone who doesn't see it."—**Me**

"Your body, your rules. Do not let society fuck you up!"—**Anna perry**

"Dear Body, you were never a problem. There is nothing wrong with your size… you're good enough already."—**Monica dunlop**

"I've finally recognized my body for what it is: a personality-delivery system, designed expressly to carry my character from place to place, now and in the years to come."
–**Anna Quindlen**

"Is "fat" really the worst thing a human being can be? Is "fat" worse than "vindictive," "jealous," "shallow," "vain," "boring," or "cruel"? Not to me." –**J.K. Rowling**

"This is it: This body is home. This is where I live and hang my hat. This is where I settle into my hips and sit easy on myself, slung together with strong muscles and bones, made gentle and forging with flesh. This body is durable, has lasted for years, hunkered down through fierce storms and allows for the peaceful erosion of age. It is like a cottage on the shore: weathered and well made, a place where a person could comfortably live. I like it here. It is my own." –**Marya Hornbacher**

"Weight loss does not make people happy. Or peaceful. Being thin does not address the emptiness that has no shape or weight or name. Even a wildly successful diet is a colossal failure

because inside the new body is the same sinking heart."
—**Geneen Roth**

"You can't eat beauty, it doesn't sustain you. What is fundamentally beautiful is compassion, for yourself and those around you. That kind of beauty inflames the heart and enchants the soul." –**Lupita Nyong'o**

"We can't hate ourselves into a version of ourselves we can love."
–**Lori Deschene**

"You have to stand up and say, 'There's nothing wrong with me or my shape or who I am; you're the one with the problem!'"
-**Jennifer Lopez**

"My limbs work, so I'm not going to complain about the way my body is shaped."—**Drew Barrymore**

"Girls of all kinds can be beautiful—from the thin, plus-sized, short, very tall, ebony to porcelain-skinned; the quirky, clumsy, shy, outgoing and all in between. It's not easy though because many people still put beauty into a confining, narrow box...think outside of the box." –**Tyra Banks**

"Beauty comes in all shapes and sizes." –**Emme**

"There is nothing more rare, nor more beautiful, than a woman being unapologetically herself; comfortable in her perfect imperfection. To me, that is the true essence of beauty." – **Steve Maraboli**

"Women who love themselves are threatening; but men who love real women, more so." – **Naomi Wolf**

"You are not a mistake. You are not a problem to be solved. But you won't discover this until you are willing to stop banging your head against the wall of shaming and caging and fearing yourself." – **Geneen Roth**

"People often say that 'beauty is in the eye of the beholder,' and I say that the most liberating thing about beauty is realizing that you are the beholder." – **Salma Hayek**

"I want to enjoy life, and I can't if I'm not eating and miserable."
-**Kate Upton**

"My body is normal, and I'm not trying to prove anything." – **Lucy Hale**

"My smile is my favorite part of my body. I think a smile can make your whole body." – **Serena William**

"I don't wanna be shaped like a girl. I love being shaped like a woman, and trust me, ladies, your man won't mind either."
-**Miley Cyrus**

"I have learned to enjoy my body when I have a few extra pounds on, just being more voluptuous." -**Fergie**

"My heart. My Body. For they are soft. I'm so done being sorry for my softness. Instead, I've grown quite fond of it" -**Sarah Nicole**

"One day I had to sit down with myself and decide that I loved myself no matter what my body looked like and what other people thought about my body." -**Gabourey Sidibe**

"I've never wanted to look like models on the cover of magazines. I represent the majority of women and I'm very proud of that." – **Adele**

"I'm not going to sacrifice my mental health to have the perfect body." -Demi Lovato
"I'm not going to conform and hurt myself and do something crazy to be a size 2." -**Amber Riley**

"Who cares if there are lumps on my thighs? I'm guilty of having human legs made up of fat, muscle, and skin, and sometimes when you sit, they get bumpy." – **Kristen Bell**

"I don't look in the mirror and go, 'Oh, I look fantastic!' Of course, I don't. Nobody is perfect. I just don't believe in perfection. But I do believe in saying, 'This is who I am and look at me not being perfect!' I'm proud of that." – **Kate Winslet**

"I would only lose weight if it affected my health or sex life, which it doesn't." -**Adele**

"I wish I could tell my younger self that she was always more than a body. She always had more to offer the world than weight loss and flat abs. So much more." – **Megan Jayne Crabbe**

"You need to be able to create a relationship with your body. Stop thinking about how other people will judge you, or other peoples opinion and find self-love first" – **Harnaam Kaur**

"We are a gorgeous, infinite circle of women of all shades, all styles, in all the ways we were made, inside of us everything blooms." -**Alicia Keys**

"My body is not yours to critique and discuss. My body is not yours for consumption. My body is my vessel. An archive of experiences. A weapon that has fought battles only I understand. A library of love, pain, struggle, victory, and mystery. Your eyes cannot define all it has endured. Do not place value upon my body, place it upon my being." – **Sophie Lewis**

"In owning the parts of me that I so badly wanted to ignore and hide, I've dismantled the shame I've held for years, and began building self acceptance for myself in its place." – **Lenea Sims**

"You don't have to fully love yourself. You just have to have that little thread of "I'm doing this for me"."- **Chelsea Charlotte**

"You don't need to be pretty like her, you can be pretty like YOU."—**Me**

"You are imperfect, permanently and inevitably flawed. And you are beautiful."
— **Amy Bloom**

"The more I like myself, the less I want to pretend to be other people." – **Jamie Lee Curtis**

| | | |
"Beauty comes in all shapes and sizes, and being a fat girl doesn't make you any less beautiful."

| | | |
"Your weight does not define your worth, your confidence and character do."

| | | |
"Don't let society's standards of beauty make you feel inferior. Embrace your curves and love yourself."

| | | |
"Being a fat girl is not a flaw, it's just a part of who you are. Embrace it and be proud of yourself."

| | | |

"Confidence is the sexiest thing a person can wear, regardless of their size."

| | | |

"There is nothing wrong with being a fat girl. It's society's narrow-mindedness that needs fixing."

| | | |

"Your body size does not determine your value as a person. You are so much more than a number on a scale."

| | | |

"Beauty has no weight limit, and it is time we start celebrating that."

| | | |

"Fat does not mean unhealthy, just as skinny does not mean healthy. Focus on being strong and taking care of yourself."
"Don't let anyone make you feel ashamed of your body. You are beautiful just the way you are."

| | | |

"You are not defined by your weight, but by your strength, resilience, and kindness."

| | | |

"Self-love is the most important kind of love. Embrace and nurture yourself, inside and out."

| | | |

"Everybody is unique in its own way. Embrace your uniqueness and let it shine." SABA QUOTES

| | | |

"You do not need to be thin to be deserving of love and happiness. You already are."

| | | |

"Your worth is not determined by your waistline. It is determined by your heart, mind, and the way you treat others."

| | | |

"Size is just a number. Focus on the things that truly matter — love, joy, and living life to the fullest."

| | | |

"Fat is not a flaw, it's just a characteristic. Embrace your body and be proud of who you are."

| | | |

"The most attractive thing about anyone is their confidence and positivity, regardless of their size."

| | | |

"Your body is your temple, and it deserves to be loved and respected, regardless of its shape or size."

| | | |

"Don't let society dictate what beauty should look like. Create your own standard of beauty and celebrate it."

| | | |

"Real beauty comes from self-acceptance and embracing your uniqueness."

| | | |

"Your worth cannot be measured by the size of your jeans. You are worthy simply because you exist."

| | | |

"It's not about fitting into society's standards – it's about loving yourself unconditionally."

| | | |

"Don't let anyone dull your sparkle. Be proud of who you are, fat or not."

That's it! I hope you enjoyed my list and use them whenever you need them. Write them on post-it notes and pin them all over your home, workspace, walls, phones, or whatever supports you best.

Chapter 5

After you graduate college it becomes harder to make friends and connections with people who are not your colleagues. But much of success is about building a network and making friends in your industry, and that involves making people like you. But how do you make friends as an adult? How do you make people like you? It seems like a subjective process, but there are universal techniques you can use to help you make small talk a bit more easily. Leaders like Warren Buffet swear by How To Win Friends And Influence People by Dale Carnegie, and the lessons of Carnegie have stood the test of time. They are classic principles in the best sense, and the fundamentals of this book are still applicable generations later. These principles do not revolve around trends or fads, they are just the building blocks of social intelligence, and how practicing good social skills can improve your life. Here are the 10 best, classic lessons we learn from Carnegie's How To Win Friends And Influence People:

1. *Do Not Criticize, Condemn or Complain*

Carnegie writes, "Any fool can criticize, condemn or complain and most fools do." He continues on to say that it takes character and self-control to be forgiving, this discipline will pay major dividends in your relationships with people.

2. *Be Generous With Praise*

Carnegie uses Schwab as an example throughout the book, as someone who exemplifies all of the tenets Carnegie preaches. Schwab used praise as the foundation of all of his relationships, "In my wide association in life, meeting with many and great people in various parts of the world," Schwab declared, "I have yet to find the person, however great or exalted in their station who did not do better work and put forth greater effort under a spirit of approval than they would ever do under a spirit of criticism."

3. *Remember Their Name*

Remembering people's names when you meet them is difficult. You casually meet a lot of people so it's challenging, but if you can train yourself to remember people's names, it makes them feel special and important. Carnegie writes, "Remember that a person's name is to that person the sweetest and most important sound in any language."

4. *Be Genuinely Interested In Other People*

Remembering a person's name, asking them questions that encourage them to talk about themselves so you discover their interests and passions are what make people believe you like them, so they in turn like you. Carnegie writes, "You make more friends in two months by becoming genuinely interested in other people than you can in two years by trying to get other people interested in you." If you break it down, you should listen 75% and only speak 25% of the time.

5. _Know The Value Of Charm_

One things people do not discuss much in the job search industry is that so much of getting an opportunity is not about talent, where you went to college or who you know, it is people liking you. A good resume may get you in the door, but charm, social skills and talent keep you there, and people will normally pick someone they enjoy being around over a candidate they don't enjoy being around as much but is more talented. Become someone people want to talk to, be genuinely interested in other people, because it will enrich your life and open so many more doors than you ever thought possible.

6. _Be Quick To Acknowledge Your Own Mistakes_

Nothing will make people less defensive and more agreeable than you being humble and reasonable enough to admit your own mistakes. Having strong and stable personal and professional relationships relies on you taking responsibility for your actions, especially your mistakes. Nothing will help end tension or a disagreement more than a swift acknowledgment and apology on your part.

7. _Don't Attempt To "Win" An Argument_

The best way to win any argument, Carnegie writes, is to avoid it.Even if you completely dismantle someone's argument with objective facts, you won't be any closer to reaching an agreement than if you made personal arguments. Carnegie cited an old saying: "A man convinced against his will/Is of the same opinion still."

8. *Begin On Common Ground*

If you are having a disagreement with someone, you start on common ground and ease your way into the difficult subjects. If you begin on polarizing ground, you'll never be able to recover, and may lose ground with subjects on which you agree.

9. *Have Others Believe Your Conclusion Is Their Own*

People can not be forced to believe anything, and persuasive people understand the power of suggestion over demand. Learn to plant the seed, and instead of telling people they're wrong, find the common ground and persuade them that what they really want is your desired outcome (obviously without telling them that is the case).

In all relationships, set boundaries.....

Chapter 6

MOST EFFECTIVE WAYS TO LOSE WEIGHT

- If you want to burn fat fast there is no getting around cardio training.
- Reduce refined carbs.
- Add fatty fish to your diet.
- Start the day with a high protein breakfast.
- Drink enough water.
- Reduce your salt intake.

All this could work but there's a lot of bad weight loss information on the internet. Much of what's recommended is questionable at best, and not based on any actual science.

However, there are several natural methods that have actually been proven to work. Here's how to get started.

1. *Add protein to your diet*

When it comes to weight loss, protein is the king of nutrients.

Your body burns calories when digesting and metabolizing the protein you eat, so a high-protein diet can boost metabolism by up to 80–100 calories per day. A high protein diet can also make you feel more full and reduce your appetite. In fact, some studies show that people eat over 400 fewer calories per day on a high-protein diet. Even something as simple as eating a high-protein breakfast (like eggs) can have a powerful effect

2. _Prioritize whole, single-ingredient foods_

One of the best things you can do to become healthier is to base your diet on whole, single-ingredient foods. By doing this, you eliminate the vast majority of added sugar, added fat, and processed food. Most whole foods are naturally very filling, making it a lot easier to keep within typical calorie limits. Eating whole foods also provides your body with the many essential nutrients that it needs to function properly. Weight loss often follows as a natural side effect of eating whole foods.

3. _Limit processed foods_

Processed foods are usually high in added sugars, added fats, and calories. What's more, processed foods are engineered to make you eat as much as possible. They're much more likely to cause addictive-like eating than unprocessed foods.

4. _Stock up on nutritious foods and snacks_

Studies have shown that the food you keep at home greatly affects weight and eating behavior. By always having nutrient-dense food available, you reduce the chances of you or other family members eating less nutritious items. There are also many nutritious snacks that are easy to prepare and take with you on the go. These include yogurt, whole fruit, nuts, carrots, and hard-boiled eggs.

5. _Limit your intake of added sugar_

Eating a lot of added sugar is linked with some of the world's leading diseases, including heart disease, type 2 diabetes, and cancer. On average, Americans eat about 15 teaspoons of added sugar each day. This amount is usually hidden in various processed foods, so you may be consuming a lot of sugar without even realizing it. Since sugar goes by many names in ingredient lists, it can be very difficult to figure out how much sugar a product actually contains. Minimizing your intake of added sugar is a great way to improve your diet.

6. _Drink water_

There's actually truth to the claim that drinking water can help with weight loss.
Drinking 0.5 liters (17 oz) of water may increase the calories you burn by 24–30% for an hour afterward. Drinking water before meals may also lead to reduced calorie intake, especially for middle-aged and older people. Water is particularly helpful for weight loss when it replaces other beverages that are high in calories and sugar..

7. _Drink (unsweetened) coffee_

Coffee is loaded with antioxidants and other beneficial compounds. Coffee drinking may support weight loss by increasing energy levels and the amount of calories you burn. Caffeinated coffee may boost your metabolism by 3–11% and reduce your risk of developing type 2 diabetes by a whopping 23–50%.

Furthermore, black coffee is very weight loss friendly, since it can make you feel full but contains almost no calories.

8. *Supplement with glucomannan*

Glucomannan is one of several weight loss pills that has been proven to work. This water-soluble, natural dietary fiber comes from the roots of the konjac plant, also known as the elephant yam. Glucomannan is low in calories, takes up space in the stomach, and delays stomach emptying. It also reduces the absorption of protein and fat, and feeds the beneficial gut bacteria.

Its exceptional ability to absorb water is believed to be what makes it so effective for weight loss. One capsule is able to turn an entire glass of water into gel.

9. *Limit liquid calories*

Liquid calories come from beverages like sugary soft drinks, fruit juices, chocolate milk, and energy drinks. These drinks can have a negative impact on your health in several ways, including an increased risk of obesity. One study showed a drastic 60% increase in the risk of obesity among children for each daily serving of a sugar-sweetened beverage. It's also important to note that your brain does not register liquid calories the same way it does solid calories, so you end up adding these calories on top of everything else that you eat.

10. *Limit your intake of refined carbs*

Refined carbs are carbs that have had most of their beneficial nutrients and fiber removed. The refining process leaves nothing but easily digested carbs, which can increase the risk of overeating and disease. The main dietary sources of refined carbs are white flour, white bread, white rice, sodas, pastries, snacks, sweets, pasta, breakfast cereals, and added sugar.

11. *Fast intermittently*

Intermittent fasting is an eating pattern that cycles between periods of fasting and eating. There are a few different ways to do intermittent fasting, including the 5:2 diet, the 16:8 method, and the eat-stop-eat method. Generally, these methods make you eat fewer calories overall, without having to consciously restrict calories during the eating periods. This should lead to weight loss, as well as numerous other health benefits.

12. *Drink (unsweetened) green*

Green tea is a natural beverage that's loaded with antioxidants. Drinking green tea is linked with many benefits, such as increased fat burning and weight loss. Green tea may increase energy expenditure by 4% and increase selective fat burning by up to 17%, especially harmful belly fat. Matcha tea is a variety of powdered green tea that may have even more powerful health benefits than regular green tea.

13. *__Eat more fruits and vegetables__*

Fruits and vegetables are extremely nutritious, weight-loss-friendly foods. In addition to being high in water, nutrients, and fiber, they usually have very low energy density. This makes it possible to eat large servings without consuming excess calories. Numerous studies have shown that people who eat more fruits and vegetables tend to weigh less.

14. *__Count calories once in a while__*

Being aware of what you're eating is very helpful when trying to lose weight. There are several effective ways to do this, including counting calories, keeping a food diary, or taking pictures of what you eat. Using an app or another electronic tool may be even more beneficial than writing in a food diary.

15. *__Try a low-carb diet__*

Many studies have shown that low-carb diets are effective for weight loss. Limiting carbs and eating more fat and protein reduces your appetite and helps you eat fewer calories. This can result in weight loss that is up to 3 times greater than that from a standard low-fat diet. A low-carb diet can also improve many risk factors for disease.

17. *__Add eggs to your diet__*

Eggs are the ultimate weight loss food. They're low in calories, high in protein, and loaded with all sorts of nutrients. High-protein foods have been shown to reduce appetite and increase fullness, compared to foods that contain less protein. Furthermore, eating eggs for breakfast may cause up to 65% greater weight loss over 8 weeks, compared to eating bagels for breakfast. It may also help you eat fewer calories throughout the rest of the day.

18. *Spice up your meals*

Chili peppers and jalapeños contain a compound called capsaicin, which may boost metabolism and increase the burning of fat. Capsaicin may also reduce appetite and calorie intake.

19. *Take probiotics*

Probiotics are live bacteria that have health benefits when eaten. They can improve digestive health and heart health, and may even help with weight loss. Studies have shown that people who are overweight and people who have obesity tend to have different gut bacteria than average-weight people, which may influence weight. Probiotics may help regulate the healthy gut bacteria. They may also block the absorption of dietary fat, while reducing appetite and inflammation. Of all the probiotic bacteria, Lactobacillus gasseri shows the most promising effects on weight loss.

20. _**Eat more fiber**_

Fiber-rich foods may help with weight loss. Foods that contain water-soluble fiber may be especially helpful, since this type of fiber can help increase the feeling of fullness. Fiber may delay stomach emptying, make the stomach expand and promote the release of satiety hormones. This can help you eat less without having to think about it. Many types of fiber can feed the friendly gut bacteria. Healthy gut bacteria have been linked with a reduced risk of obesity. Just make sure to increase your fiber intake gradually to avoid abdominal discomfort, such as bloating, cramps, and diarrhea.

21. _**Brush your teeth after meals**_

Many people brush or floss their teeth or use mouthwash after eating. Dental hygiene products can temporarily affect the taste of food and beverages, which may help limit the desire to snack or eat between meals.

22. _**Work to overcome food addiction**_

Food addiction involves overpowering cravings and changes in your brain chemistry that make it harder to resist eating certain foods. This is a major cause of overeating for many people, and affects a significant percentage of the population. In fact, a recent 2014 study found that almost 20% of people fulfilled the criteria for food addiction. Some foods are much more likely to cause symptoms of addiction than others. This includes highly processed junk foods that are high in sugar, fat, or both. Consulting with a healthcare professional can help.

23. Do some sort of cardio
Doing cardio whether it's jogging, running, cycling, power walking, or hiking is a great way to burn calories and improve both mental and physical health. Cardio has been shown to improve many risk factors for heart disease. It can also help reduce body weight. Cardio seems to be particularly effective at reducing the fat that builds up around your organs and causes metabolic disease.

24. *Add resistance exercises*

Loss of muscle mass is a common side effect of dieting. If you lose a lot of muscle, your body will start burning fewer calories than before. Resistance exercises, like lifting weights, can help prevent this loss in muscle mass.

25. *Use whey protein*

Most people get enough protein from diet alone. However, for those who don't, taking a whey protein supplement is an effective way to boost protein intake. One study shows that replacing part of your calories with whey protein can cause significant weight loss, while also increasing lean muscle mass. Just make sure to read the ingredients list, because some varieties are loaded with sugar and other additives.

26. Practice mindful eating

Mindful eating is a method used to increase awareness while eating. It helps you make conscious food choices and develop awareness of your hunger and satiety cues. It then helps you eat well in response to those cues. Mindful eating has been shown to have significant effects on weight, eating behavior, and stress in individuals who have obesity. It's especially helpful against binge eating and emotional eating. By making conscious food choices, increasing your awareness, and listening to your body, weight loss should follow.

28. ***Focus on changing your lifestyle***

Dieting is one of those things that almost always fails in the long term. In fact, people who "diet" tend to gain more weight over time. Instead of focusing only on losing weight, make it a primary goal to nourish your body with nutritious food and daily movement. there's been a rising interest in body positivity as a movement. What better way to celebrate this movement than by creating a post with all the most impactful and inspiring quotes? 50 Quotes for body positivity, self-esteem, and body image which are so helpful when I'm struggling with body image issues or am looking to boost my self-esteem. These inspiring quotes can be just the kick-start we sometimes need to feel better about ourselves.

Chapter 7

FINAL WORDS

When your friend or loved one announces they are trying to lose weight, how should you respond? What you say can make a difference in their success. Support Makes a Difference in Weight Loss Success. Your support can make a big difference to someone who is trying to lose weight. People who have support find it easier to stick to a weight loss plan and are more likely to meet their weight loss goals.

If you know someone who is trying to lose weight, you can support them by:

- ☐ choosing your words carefully, focusing on positivity and encouragement.
- ☐ listening without judgment.
- ☐ modeling healthy behaviors in your own life.
- ☐ letting them know you think they are amazing no matter their weight.
- ☐ offering to support them in any way they need.
- ☐ No matter what weight loss program your friend or loved one is following, your support and encouragement will make a difference in their long-term success.

And by saying this few things:

<u>*Supportive Things You Can Say to Someone Trying to Lose Weight*</u>

- "It's wonderful that you're focusing on your health." Shift the focus away from weight. Instead, compliment their efforts towards better health and wellness. This shows that you see the bigger picture and you want to support them as they create a healthier lifestyle.

- "How can I support you?" The best way to know how to support someone with their weight loss goals is to simply ask. They may want a workout buddy, or they might just want someone to talk to when they face challenges. Some people even prefer it if you don't mention diet or weight at all.

- "Let's get salads tonight." Be sensitive to their new dietary needs. Don't suggest pizza when you know they are trying to avoid it. Instead, suggest a restaurant with ample healthy options, or better yet, let them pick.

- "You look great!" It's better to give a general compliment that they are looking terrific rather than specifically saying they look skinny or that you can tell they've lost weight. Encouraging words that are not about body size can help people lose more weight. Choose words that show you think your friend or loved one is amazing, no matter their size.

- "Do you want to go on a walk with me?" Suggest things you can do together that aren't focused on food. Invite them to join you in any fitness activities you enjoy, such as going for a walk, joining a group exercise class, or playing tennis. Sharing time to exercise together will increase the intensity and duration of both your workouts.

Don't ever say this to them:

Things You Shouldn't Say to Someone Trying to Lose Weight

- "You look great now. You don't need to lose weight." You might think this is a compliment, but you shouldn't assume someone is trying to lose weight because they want to look better. Many people are perfectly happy with the way they look at any weight.

- N"Let's grab some fast food!" People often eat similar amounts and types of foods as the people they're eating with, so try to make healthy choices and keep your portion sizes reasonable when snacking or dining with your friend. Better yet, remove food as the focus of your time together and invite them to join you for other activities.

- "I know someone that lost 50 pounds on a special diet." Don't offer anecdotes about people you know who succeeded or failed on popular or fad diet plans. First, this invites comparison which isn't helpful for someone embarking on a weight loss journey. Second, you should leave any diet advice to the experts. Many popular diets have contradictory guidelines, which can be confusing to someone trying a new eating plan. Some diets can even be dangerous for people with certain medical histories.

- "Should you really be eating that?" Unless this person has specifically asked you to hold them accountable for everything they put in their mouth, don't take on the role of food police. This can be embarrassing and discouraging to someone trying to change their eating habits. Playing food police can even lead to worse dietary choices rather than better ones. Negative messages about foods and food choices can lead dieters to eat significantly more unhealthy snacks.

- "One bite won't hurt." On the other end of the spectrum, don't try to entice the person to have food that isn't healthy or on their plan. One little bite can hurt them, especially if they are trying to overcome binge eating disorder or have other medical conditions. One little bite often leads to more, and having an unplanned "cheat meal" can undo a lot of hard work.

- "How much do you weigh?" Some people are more sensitive about disclosing their weight than others, so it's always best not to ask someone their weight. If they want to share it, they will volunteer it themselves. Remember that the number on the scale isn't always the best measure of progress towards better health.

Always remember:

Your body is fantastic. Appreciate every part of your body because it's yours. Explore a list of body love quotes that are sure to inspire self-love.

Your uniqueness shines through every inch of your skin.
A body glows because of the amazing spirit held within.
Everything about you is unique. Embrace it.
Respect and love your body just the way it is.
Only you can define beauty. Consider yourself fabulous.
Your body is a precious gift. Show it the love it deserves.
When you love your body, you project self-confidence.
Let your eyes shine with love and adoration when you look at yourself.
Love your body the way it loves you.
Your body contains the precious person within it. Cherish it.
Sometimes it can be challenging to embrace all the unique aspects of your body. But acceptance and love are the first steps on the road to a positive you. Appreciate every part of your body and smile brightly at the fabulous body that houses your unique self.

Give your body the love and respect it deserves.
Much like a flower, everybody blooms a bit differently. But they are all glorious.
Appreciate the uniqueness of your body.
Be confident in your own skin. It makes you sparkle.
You are powerful. You are strong. Be confident in your body.
Build a powerful body image one positive thought at a time.
Shout out to you for loving your body.
Your body is where you live. You set the rules.
Embrace your body, and confidence blooms.
Post a self-love caption on Instagram. Show off your body in all its glory with a short and sweet message. It's essential to love the skin you're in.

Show your body some love.
Loving your body is the best trend.
Be proud of your body.
Take a moment to fall in love with your body.
Pride in your body looks great on you.
A positive body image makes a mind happy.
Smile and show your confidence.
Acceptance is a beautiful thing.
Love every part of yourself.
Tell yourself only kind words.

Embrace Your Body Quotes for Body Confidence
Filled with happiness and positive vibes
Image Credit

Once you embrace your body, you find beautiful things to love about yourself. You get strength from appreciating, accepting, and loving just how unique you are. Nourish your soul with a confidence-boosting quote.

If the world is a house, your body is your home. Love it.
Your body is a glorious piece of art. Every detail makes it stand out.
The beauty of your soul radiates through your eyes.
It's all the pieces of you that make you extraordinary.
Be comfortable with every part of yourself, and embrace your entire being.
Cherish the divine beauty of the artwork that is your body.
The charm of your soul shines like a beacon through every inch of your skin.
Feel good about yourself. You are worth it.
Allow your exceptional qualities to shine with pride. Love your body.
Loving yourself takes work. But you are worth it. Love the artistry that is you.

Each body is special, memorable, and beautiful. There is a greatness inside of you that will not be tamed. Embrace how exceptional you are, inside and out.

Your body is the ship guiding your journey through life. Love it with all your heart.
When you remind yourself daily how much you love your body, you believe it.

Find happiness by loving your body, mind, and soul.

Loving your body brings more positivity and grace to your life.

Take a moment every day to appreciate and cherish the body that's uniquely yours.

Be proud of your body. It's an amazing home for your spirit.

Live for this moment by loving the vessel that carries you.

Accepting yourself is the first step to moving forward toward body positivity.

Everything about your body is unique and special. Show it the love.

Hold your head high so your crown stays on that beautiful body.

Loving your body fills your soul with confidence.

Love Your Body Messages to Share

Confidence is built one positive thought at a time. Use these unique quotes to promote body positivity and love in your friend circle. Add them to a tumbler or shirt to remind yourself how wonderful your body is. Create a card for a friend who might be struggling with body image issues. These quotes also work as wall decals to spread positivity, love, and acceptance in your home. It's important to remind yourself how special your body is each and every day.